Storing up problems

The medical case for a slimmer nation

REPORT OF A WORKING PARTY   2004

Royal College of
Physicians

Royal College of Paediatrics
& Child Health

Faculty of
Public Health

Royal College of Physicians of London
11 St Andrews Place, London NW1 4LE
www.rcplondon.ac.uk
Registered Charity No 210508

Royal College of Paediatrics & Child Health
50 Hallam Street, London W1W 6DE
www.rcpch.ac.uk
Registered Charity No 1057744

Faculty of Public Health
4 St Andrews Place, London NW1 4LE
www.fphm.org.uk
Registered Charity No 263894

ISBN 1 86016 200 2

Cover photograph: CRISTINA PEDRAZZINI/SCIENCE PHOTO LIBRARY
Typeset by Dan-Set Graphics, Telford, Shropshire
Printed in Great Britain by Sarum ColourView Group, Salisbury, Wiltshire

Contents

Members of the Working Party

Peter Kopelman MD FRCP (*Chair*)
Vice-Principal and Professor of Clinical Medicine,
Barts and The London, Queen Mary's School of Medicine and Dentistry,
University of London

Fiona Adshead MBBS MRCP(UK) FFPH
Policy Advisor, Faculty of Public Health; Director of Public Health,
Camden Primary Care Trust, London

Arran Elkeles MA Chartered FCIPD
Legal Consultant, Aikin Driver Partnership, London

Penny Gibson FRCP FRCPCH
Advisor on Childhood Obesity, Royal College of Paediatrics and Child
Health; Consultant Paediatrician, Blackwater Valley and Hart Primary
Care Trust

Ian Gilmore MD FRCP
Registrar, Royal College of Physicians

Catherine Law OBE MD FRCP FRCPCH FFPH
Reader in Children's Health, Institute of Child Health, University College
London

Alan Maryon Davis MRCP(UK) FFPH FRIPH
Director of Public Health, Southwark; Senior Lecturer in Public Health,
King's College London

Chloe Underwood PhD
Head of Policy and Communications, Faculty of Public Health, London

Advisor

Paul Lincoln Hon MFPH
Chief Executive, National Heart Forum, London

Acknowledgements

The Working Party acknowledges the advice of members of a specially convened think tank which gave impetus for this report. Those who participated included representatives from government and government agencies; the medical profession; health service management; education; advertising; and food manufacturing and distribution.

The Working Party acknowledges with sincere thanks the work of Joanna Reid of the RCP Publications Department for her skill in helping to draft the report and editing the final text, and the dedication of other members of the Department who have enabled the publication of the report within a very short timescale.

Foreword

We must not underestimate the threat to millions of people who are overweight or obese.

Being overweight restricts body activity, damages health and shortens life; and it harms self-esteem and social life. Heart disease, stroke, joint problems and the commonest form of diabetes are direct effects of overweight and obesity. The harm to individuals from childhood onwards is only too evident in the NHS, both in numbers of patients affected and in the costs of health and social care.

The purpose of this report is to bring the concerns of the medical profession and public health specialists to the attention of government, local authorities, health professionals in all disciplines, educators, food manufacturers, retailers, advertisers and the public. The report identifies factors that contribute to the relentless increase in obesity in our society; and highlights ways of halting and reversing it.

Our recommendations are principally aimed at government and policy makers. They are in a key position to do something about the underlying causes – through education, persuasion, policy and direction. But we all have a role to play.

Failure to act now will have severe consequences for millions of individuals, for the nation's health and for the health service.

February 2004

Professor Carol Black
President, Royal College of Physicians

Professor Alan Craft
President, Royal College of Paediatrics and Child Health

Professor Siân Griffiths
President, Faculty of Public Health

Recommendations

We are concerned about the serious social and health penalties that the nation is paying as a consequence of the increasing rates of overweight and obesity among the population. This report highlights the importance of immediate and sustained action. The recommendations are directed at central government but they also require implementation in every locality, together with an understanding of the social and cultural factors that are behind the progressive increase in overweight and obesity. The recommendations apply to all age groups from childhood through to old age, and specifically include people who are at particular risk, whether disadvantaged or on a low income, and those from ethnic groups who are at greater medical risk from increased body weight.

1 **A cross-governmental task force should be established at Cabinet level to develop national strategies for tackling the threat from overweight and obesity, and to oversee the implementation of these strategies.**

In order to convert the strategies proposed by the task force into measurable outcomes, it is particularly important that its remit includes implementation as well as policy goals, and that it sets milestones for their achievement. The task force should have senior ministerial involvement and fully engage government departments with responsibilities that include health, education, fiscal policies, transport, food and agriculture, sport and culture, and Europe. The task force will drive a new public health initiative that engages the public, public services, local government, schools, the voluntary sector, industry and business. Specific priorities for the task force will be the promotion of healthy lifestyles for children and young people. *(Chapters 2, 3, 4 and 5)*

2 **Government should mount a sustained public education campaign to improve people's understanding of the benefits of healthy eating and active living, and to motivate people to eat a healthier diet and adopt a more active lifestyle.**

The campaign should be directed at everyone, whatever their background, but should particularly aim to engage children, young people, disadvantaged people and those from ethnic groups at increased risk from increasing fatness. The campaign would aim to bring about a cultural shift in public attitudes towards the type and amount of food eaten and the importance of regular physical activity. *(Chapters 3 and 4)*

3 **New standards in nutritional content, food labelling, and food marketing and promotion should be agreed jointly by the food industry and the Food Standards Agency. Incentives to encourage the production, promotion and sale of healthier foods should be introduced.**

Children should be protected by introducing effective control, and legislation if necessary, over the marketing of food and drink with high fat and/or sugar content. The Food Standards Agency should work with the food industry to develop good practice in marketing and to implement a simple food labelling scheme, with clear and easily recognisable symbols indicating nutritional and calorie content, in accordance with European Union proposals. Food manufacturers and processors should develop a wider range of lower-calorie alternatives, introduce stepped reductions in fat and sugar content in existing products, and actively promote these foods through marketing, promotional campaigns and pricing strategies. Food producers and retailers should stimulate demand for fresh fruit and vegetables, leaner meat and fish, through more vigorous and imaginative marketing. Tax and other fiscal measures should be considered as a means of encouraging the production, promotion and sale of healthier foods. *(Chapters 3 and 4)*

4 **Population-wide initiatives should be implemented at local level to tackle obesity. Public services should take the lead by promoting healthy eating and increased physical activity in public places and institutions, such as schools and hospitals.**

Local action plans should include initiatives aimed at priority target groups in a variety of settings such as home, school, workplace and primary care. Consideration should be given to incorporating a whole-school approach to healthy eating and physical activity within the statutory schools inspection framework. Strategies should be adopted to reduce the dependency on car use and to increase opportunities for walking, cycling, using stairs and other active forms of recreation and transport. All planning applications and public policies should require an assessment/prediction of health impact, and encourage the incorporation of features to support healthy eating and physical activity. Consideration should be given to the setting up of annual national award schemes for the best examples of good practice in tackling obesity at local level. *(Chapters 3 and 4)*

5   The prevention and management of overweight and obesity should be included in all NHS plans, policies and clinical care strategies. Appropriate training programmes for doctors, nurses and other health professionals should be established.

The prevention and management of overweight and obesity must be incorporated within NHS policies, including clinical governance, and integrated into programmes for the prevention and management of chronic diseases. All undergraduate and postgraduate training must include detailed instruction about the promotion of healthy eating and an active lifestyle. The medical royal colleges and other health professional academic bodies should press for expansion of the nutrition and physical activity elements in undergraduate, postgraduate and professional education and training. *(Chapters 4 and 5)*

6   There should be further funded research to improve understanding of the societal and cultural factors behind the epidemic of overweight and obesity, and the development and implementation of effective prevention and treatments.

The evidence base on the causes of obesity and the health benefits and cost-effectiveness of prevention and treatments should be expanded. *(Chapters 3, 4 and 5)*

Guiding principles for implementing the recommendations.

▶ Concentrate on solutions not problems – with an emphasis on action to create health-promoting environments.

▶ Be long-term and sustainable, recognising that behaviour change is complex, difficult and takes time.

▶ Engage the whole community – healthy weight is everybody's business.

▶ Help those in most need and close the health gap between different population groups resulting from geography, ethnicity and socio-economic status.

▶ Promote the positive benefits of healthy eating, active living and healthy weight.

▶ Avoid 'victim-blaming' which creates its own problems of guilt, stigma, alienation and bullying.

▶ Empower and assist individuals and groups to take action according to their own opportunities and responsibilities.

Adapted from: *Overweight and obesity guidelines*. Australia: National Health and Medical Research Council, 2003. www.nhmrc.gov.au/media/rel2003/obese.htm

Glossary

Apnoea: temporary cessation of breathing.

Arterial thrombosis: formation of blood clots in the arteries (blood vessels).

Atherosclerosis: generalised hardening of the walls of the arteries.

Blood pressure: the pressure created by blood pumped out of the heart and passing through the arteries of the body.

Body mass index (BMI): a measure of body fatness that takes account of both body weight and height. It is expressed as body weight (kg) divided by the square of height (m^2).

Cardiovascular: cardiovascular refers to the whole circulatory system: the heart, the arteries and veins of the body and the arteries and veins of the lungs.

Central/abdominal obesity: fat tissue that is localised around the lower trunk/abdominal region.

Cholesterol: a fatty substance in the bloodstream; high levels are associated with an increased risk of heart attack and stroke.

Cirrhosis: a disease of the liver in which normal tissue is replaced by fibrous or scar tissue.

Comorbidity: associated disease or illness.

Coronary heart disease (CHD): abnormalities of the blood vessels supplying blood to the heart muscle. This can result in angina or heart attacks.

Deep vein thrombosis: formation of blood clot(s) in veins that lie deeply within the body, particularly in the legs.

Diabetes type 2: an abnormal rise in blood sugar levels as a consequence of impaired insulin action.

Diaphragm: the internal muscular partition separating the abdomen from the chest.

Endometrium: the inner lining of the womb.

Fibrosis: the formation of fibrous or scar tissue.

Gastro-oesophageal reflux: regurgitation of stomach contents into the lower portion of the gullet.

Health inequalities: differences in health and access to healthcare for different groups within a society.

Heart failure: congestion in the lungs and dependent parts of the body that results from the impaired pumping action of the chambers of the heart.

Hiatus hernia: displacement of part of the stomach from the abdomen into the chest cavity, through the opening in the diaphragm through which the oesophagus (gullet) passes.

Hyperlipidaemic: having high levels of blood fats.

Hypertension: high blood pressure.

In utero: in the womb.

Nutrient: a substance that provides nourishment for the body and promotes its growth and repair. Essential nutrients include proteins, carbohydrates, fats and oils, minerals, vitamins, and water.

Obesity: a disease in which excess body fat has accumulated to an extent that health may be adversely affected. It is defined by a body mass index greater than 30.

Osteoarthritis: 'wear and tear' problems of joints, with changes in cartilage and bone.

Osteoporosis: thinning and weakening of the bones, which occurs mostly in older people, especially women. It affects the whole skeleton but most commonly causes fractures in the wrist, spine and hip.

Vascular disease: disease of the blood vessels usually characterised by 'hardening' of the blood vessel wall.

1 Introduction

1.1 Overweight and obesity are now major causes of preventable health problems in the UK. In England, they affect more than half the adult population and involve people of every age, every region and from all population groups. The rise in the prevalence of overweight and obesity has extremely serious implications, not only for individual health, but also for the nation's health and for the economy. As this report amply demonstrates, the health problems caused by excess weight lead to a wide range of debilitating and life-threatening conditions, including cardiovascular disease, type 2 diabetes, stroke, cancers, osteoarthritis, liver and gall bladder disease, and respiratory and musculoskeletal problems. In addition, obesity may lower self-esteem, lead to social discrimination and contribute to mental illness. The stark reality is that overweight and obese people die prematurely.

1.2 In 1962, the Royal College of Physicians published a report that made a seminal contribution to public health in the UK, *Smoking and health*.[1] The fundamental description of the dangers of smoking-related diseases and the promotion of tobacco products remains unchallenged. The report's contribution to the change in smoking prevalence since 1962 has been estimated to have saved about 1.6 million lives. It is not correct, or appropriate, to draw exact parallels between cigarette smoking and obesity. Nevertheless, similarities do exist between the social influences that persuaded previous (and current) generations to smoke cigarettes and the current social environment which encourages overeating and lack of exercise. Also, in terms of effects, both these modern lifestyle 'diseases' not only cause serious illness but also substantially shorten life expectancy (see Chapter 2). The advent of type 2 diabetes in young people – a condition which shortens life but was traditionally confined to adults – is a clear signal of the immediacy of the threat from overweight and obesity to public health in the early part of the twenty-first century.

1.3 Recent reports have emphasised the challenge to public health from overweight and obesity. One from the National Audit Office (NAO), *Tackling obesity in England*,[2] calculated the substantial human cost and serious financial consequences for the National Health Service and the economy, and made a number of important recommendations that have been partly addressed by government. More recently, there has been a Parliamentary Inquiry into obesity that will report in 2004. The latter report, in line with the NAO, is likely to make recommendations on a wide range of issues, including the role of the NHS and healthcare professionals. The present report has therefore focused on the medical consequences of obesity and on measures for prevention and health promotion. These are not easy problems to tackle. The immediate major challenge is to halt the upward trend in the prevalence of obesity and to raise public awareness that even modest weight loss confers significant benefit (Chapter 3). Although the strategies adopted for prevention or control must be culturally appropriate and sensitive to the self-esteem and behaviour of those affected, they must of necessity challenge social influences and be responsive to changes over time (Chapter 4).

1.4   The Chief Medical Officer for England has identified overweight and obesity as a priority for action.[3] He recognised that the Department of Health cannot tackle obesity alone and confirmed that, despite actions being taken across government, more needs to be done to improve diet and increase physical activity. He recommended that the food industry should be 'strongly encouraged' to ensure that consumers are able to make informed choices about the sugar, fat and salt content of foods, and developed a case for the 'precautionary principle' in the marketing of foods to children. In addition, he encouraged local government 'to review the [physical activity] facilities provided in their areas addressing the needs for all'.

1.5   The recommendations of the present report have taken these issues further – the medical case for tackling overweight and obesity is so compelling that immediate and concerted action must be taken. Medical intervention alone is not enough. The prevention of diseases caused by overweight and obesity will only be achieved, as we have recommended, by an effective comprehensive strategy organised across many fronts.

References

1   Royal College of Physicians. *Smoking and health.* London: RCP, 1962.
2   National Audit Office. *Tackling obesity in England.* Report by the Comptroller and Auditor General. Norwich: The Stationery Office, 2001.
3   Department of Health. *Annual Report of the Chief Medical Officer 2002.* London: DH, 2002.

2 The obesity time bomb: its impact and consequences

2.1   Overweight and obesity are now so common among the world's population that they are beginning to replace undernutrition and infectious diseases as the most significant contributors to ill health.[1] The National Audit Office estimated for England that each year 30,000 excess deaths result from obesity,[2] constituting 6% of all deaths. Moreover, many of these people die prematurely. However, despite the compelling evidence, many people, including doctors, continue to consider obesity as a self-inflicted condition of little medical significance.

Box 2.1 Definitions and measures of overweight and obesity.

Definition
Obesity is a disorder in which excess body fat has accumulated to an extent that health may be adversely affected.

Measures
▶ The most widely used measure of body fatness is currently body mass index (BMI), defined as a person's weight in kilograms divided by the square of their height in metres.
▶ Obesity is defined as a BMI of 30 (kg/m^2) or more.
▶ Overweight is defined as a BMI between 25 and 29.9.
▶ BMI cut-off values are ethnic-dependent and appear to be lower in certain populations: a BMI of 27.5 or more in an Asian person is associated with comparable morbidities to those seen in a Caucasian person with a BMI of 30.[3]
▶ Additional information about health risks is given by waist circumference, with greater waist circumference indicating increased abdominal fat and carrying increased health risks.
▶ In children, BMI varies greatly with age. Definitions of obesity and overweight therefore depend on comparison with age- and gender-specific standards.

Increasing prevalence

2.2   There has been a rapid increase in the prevalence of overweight and obesity in all age groups across the UK over the last 20 years. For example, according to the latest Health Survey for England (2002),[4] between 1993 and 2002 the proportion of overweight and obese adults rose from 62% to 70% among men, and from 56% to 63% among women. So, over two-thirds of men and nearly two-thirds of women were either overweight or obese in 2002. The proportion who were categorised as obese increased from 13% of men in 1993 to 22% in 2002, and from 16% of women in 1993 to 23% in 2002. Obesity now affects over one in five adults in the UK.

Box 2.2 Obesity in England, 1980–2002. Some summary facts.[4–6]

▶ Obesity in 2- to 4-year-old children almost doubled (5%–9%) in 10 years (1989–1998).

▶ Obesity in 6- to 15-year-olds trebled (5%–16%) in 11 years (1990–2001).

▶ Obesity in adult women nearly trebled (8%–23%) in 22 years (1980–2002).

▶ Obesity in adult men nearly quadrupled (6%–22%) in 22 years (1980–2002).

2.3   In 1992 the then Government set targets in the *Health of the nation*[7] for a reduction in the prevalence of obesity in adult men and women by 2005 to the rates recorded in 1980 – 6% for men and 8% for women. However, far from reducing in prevalence, current high obesity rates are set to escalate at an alarming pace.

2.4   Overweight young people have a 50% chance of being overweight adults, and children of overweight parents have twice the risk of being overweight compared to those with healthy weight parents. Obese 10- to 14-year-olds with at least one obese parent have a 79% chance of becoming obese adults.[8] Furthermore, parental obesity more than doubles the risk of adult obesity in obese and non-obese children under 10 years.

2.5   If current trends continue, *at least* one-third of adults, one-fifth of boys and one-third of girls will be obese by 2020 (Figs 2.1 and 2.2). These forward projections from existing data are conservative. If the rapid acceleration in childhood obesity in the last decade is taken into account, the predicted prevalence in children for 2020 will be in excess of 50%.

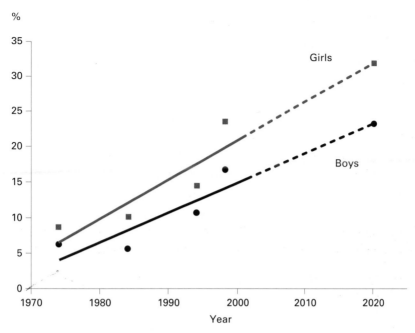

Fig 2.1 The escalating obesity rates in children in England[9] (reproduced with permission from the International Obesity Task Force).

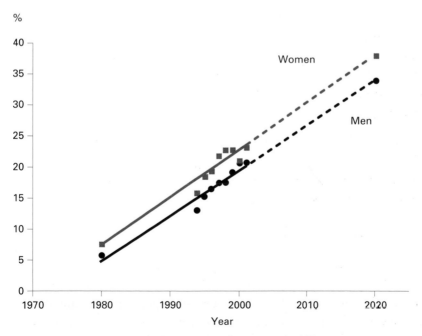

Fig 2.2 The escalating obesity rates in adults in England[4,10] (reproduced with permission from the International Obesity Task Force).

Social patterns

2.6   Excess body weight affects all social groups but is more common in
lower socio-economic and socially disadvantaged groups, particularly among
women. The Chief Medical Officer (CMO) for England noted, in his Annual
Report for 2002,[11] that 14% of men and women in professional groups were
obese compared to 19% of men and 28% of women in unskilled manual
occupations[6] (see also Para 3.18). There are also important differences in
prevalence and health consequences of overweight and obesity between
ethnic groups. In England in 1999, the prevalence of obesity among Black
Caribbean women was 50% higher than average and among Pakistani
women 25% higher than average. Obesity in Asian children was almost four
times more common than in white children.[11]

Effects of nutrition on fetal development

2.7   There is evidence that undernutrition of the mother (and consequently,
the fetus) during pregnancy may determine the later onset of obesity, hypertension and type 2 diabetes, independent of any genetic inheritance. The proposed explanation for this is that an adverse nutritional environment *in utero*
may cause defects in the development of body organs leading to 'programmed'
susceptibility. This susceptibility interacts with later diet and environmentally
induced stresses to cause overt diseases many decades later. For example,
alterations in pancreatic islet cell function during fetal development will
increase the likelihood of type 2 diabetes developing later.[12]

2.8   This may be relevant when considering the relationship between
excess weight and social class/ethnic group and its impact on health.

How overweight and obesity damage health: the medical case for a slimmer nation

2.9   The health consequences of overweight and obesity are wide ranging
and serious.[13] At present, overweight and obesity may be more common in
older age groups but the increase in the proportion of overweight and obese
children is of major medical concern. The medical complications from
overweight and obesity may become evident throughout life but are likely to
occur much earlier because of the increasing fatness of children and young
people. As well as exacerbating many health problems, increasing degrees of
fatness shorten life (see Para 2.15).

Research evidence 1: early death

In the Framingham Heart Study, the risk of a premature death increased by 1% for each extra pound (0.45 kg) increase in weight between the ages of 30 years and 42 years, and by 2% for each pound between the ages of 50 years and 62 years.[14]

Distribution of fat

2.10 Increasing body fatness is accompanied by profound changes in the way the body works. These changes are partly dependent upon where fat is placed or distributed around the body. *Generalised obesity* (fat distributed around the whole body) results in alterations in the blood circulation and heart function, while *central/abdominal obesity* (fatness mainly around the chest and abdomen) restricts chest movements and alters breathing function. Fat around the abdomen is also a major contributor to the development of diabetes, hypertension, and alterations in blood lipid (fat and cholesterol) concentrations.

Overweight and obesity in children and young people[15]

2.11 The most common immediate consequences of overweight and obesity in childhood are social and psychological. Negative stigma and bullying can contribute to low self-esteem and depression, and may have a significant effect on future mental and physical health.

2.12 Childhood overweight is also associated with increased risk factors for heart disease such as raised blood pressure, blood cholesterol and blood sugar. Indeed, most, if not all, the medical complications seen in adulthood may begin their manifestation in overweight young people.

2.13 The most significant long-term consequence of obesity in childhood is its persistence into adulthood. Childhood obesity that continues into adult life not only increases the adult risk of disease due to obesity but also its occurrence at an earlier age. Obese adults who were overweight as adolescents have higher levels of weight-related ill health and a higher risk of early death than adults who only became obese in adulthood.

Type 2 diabetes

2.14 Of great concern is the appearance of type 2 diabetes in children and adolescents, with its potential to lead to later complications of heart disease, stroke, amputation of a limb due to vascular disease and/or infection, kidney failure and blindness (see also Para 2.16).[16]

Research evidence 2: type 2 diabetes in children and young people

A long-term study of 51 Canadian patients aged 18–33 years, diagnosed with type 2 diabetes before the age of 17 years, showed that seven had died; three others were on dialysis; one became blind at the age of 26; and one had had a toe amputation. Of 56 pregnancies in this cohort, only 35 had resulted in live births (62.5%).[17]

Health consequences

Early death

2.15   The risk of early death from all disease-related causes, including cancers and cardiovascular disease, is increased by overweight and obesity.[18,19] Excess weight is associated with major decreases in life expectancy. Moreover, the combined effect of smoking and obesity is additive, almost doubling the number of years of life lost.[20]

Research evidence 3: early death

Analysis of prospective findings in the Framingham Heart Study showed that 40-year-old women, who were non-smokers, lost 3.3 years of expected life because of overweight (BMI 25–29.9), and men of similar age lost 3.1 years. Forty-year-old non-smoking obese women (BMI 30 or over) lost 7.1 years of life because of obesity, and obese men of comparable status lost 6.7 years. However, in obese people who smoked, the years of life lost almost doubled: obese female smokers lost 13.3 years of expected life and obese male smokers lost 13.7 years of life, compared to life expectancy for normal weight non-smoking women and men. BMI at ages 30 to 49 years predicted mortality after ages 50 to 69 years, even after adjustment for BMI at age 50 to 69 years.[20]

The American Cancer Society's Prevention Study, of over 62,000 men and 260,000 women who had never smoked, showed that the higher the subjects' BMI (from moderate degrees of overweight to obesity), the greater their risk of premature death from all causes, including cardiovascular disease and cancer. The relative risk associated with increased BMI was highest among men and women aged 30 to 44 years and declined after the age of 75 years.[19]

Diabetes

2.16   Increasing fatness is closely associated with the development of type 2 diabetes. This type of diabetes used to be diagnosed in middle to later life, but is now increasingly seen in young adults and children (see Para 2.14). Type 2 diabetes is characterised by a resistance to the action of insulin, the hormone that regulates blood sugar levels, rather than a deficiency of insulin (type 1 diabetes). There is concern that diabetic complications may arise earlier in adult life in those acquiring diabetes in childhood or adolescence.

Research evidence 4: type 2 diabetes

Prospective population studies confirm a close link between increasing body fatness and type 2 diabetes. In the Nurses Cohort Study in the USA, BMI was the most important predictor of the risk of diabetes: in the female nurses, the risk of diabetes was increased five-fold for those with a BMI over 25, and 93-fold for those with a BMI of 35 or more.[21] Similarly, the risk of diabetes in men increases for all BMI levels of 24 or above.[22] The risk of diabetes, adjusted for age, is 42-fold higher in men with a BMI of 35 or more.

The effect on the heart

2.17   Increased fatness affects the heart and its function, because the heavier the body is the more oxygen it demands. The amount of blood in the body increases, putting an abnormal workload on the heart, which leads eventually to adverse structural changes of the heart. This in turn can lead to raised blood pressure.

2.18   Additionally, excess weight increases the risk of coronary heart disease (CHD).

Research evidence 5: heart failure

In the Framingham Heart Study, increased BMI (25 or greater) was associated with an increased risk of heart failure. In obese subjects (BMI 30 or greater), the risk was double that of normal weight subjects.[23]

Research evidence 6: coronary heart disease

In the Nurses Cohort Study, the risk of CHD increased two-fold for women with a BMI of 25–28.9 and 3.6-fold for a BMI above 29.[24] In the Framingham Heart Study, the 26-year incidence of CHD in women and men was proportionately related to excess weight: the incidence of CHD increased 2.4-fold in obese women and two-fold in obese men under the age of 50 years.[14]

Haemostasis

2.19   The haemostatic, or clotting, system plays an important role in the development of atherosclerosis ('hardened' arteries), and associated vascular complications. Obesity is associated with increased 'stickiness' or coagulability of the blood. It therefore clots more easily, increasing the risk of arterial and deep vein thrombosis.[25–28]

Research evidence 7: haemostasis

Plasminogen activator inhibitor-1 (PAI-1) is the main natural inhibitor of fibrinolysis or breakdown of fibrin (blood clots). As PAI-1 levels increase, there is a greater tendency for fibrin to accumulate. Fat tissue appears to be an important source of PAI-1 and is responsible for elevated concentrations in obese subjects; as body fat increases so does PAI-1 production.[27] High concentrations of PAI-1 favour the development of atherosclerosis and its acute complications.

Blood lipids

2.20   Overweight and obesity are associated with detrimental changes in blood lipid (fat) concentrations that are recognised risk factors for the development of CHD (Box 2.3).

Box 2.3 Changes in blood lipid concentrations associated with obesity.

▶ Increase in total cholesterol
▶ Increased triglycerides and low-density lipoproteins
▶ Reduced high-density lipoprotein (HDL) cholesterol.

Metabolic syndrome

2.21   In clinical practice, central obesity is frequently accompanied by the development of type 2 diabetes, alterations in blood lipids, and raised blood pressure. The cluster of these factors, which predisposes to the early development of CHD and premature death, is recognised as the metabolic syndrome.[29] Childhood obesity is a powerful predictor of metabolic syndrome in early adulthood.

Research evidence 8: metabolic syndrome

In North America, the prevalence of the metabolic syndrome in adults with central obesity who take no exercise is approximately 25%. Several cohort studies have confirmed that central obesity is associated with greater cardiovascular morbidity and mortality than generalised obesity.[30–32]

Breathing abnormalities during sleep

2.22   Obese children and adults are at risk of disordered breathing during sleep. Such abnormalities are probably under-recognised and may lead to daytime sleepiness and/or headaches. An increased amount of fat in the chest wall and abdomen alters the mechanical properties of the chest and the diaphragm. This leads to changes in breathing patterns, reduced lung volume and altered patterns of ventilation to each lung region. Increased fatness also makes it harder to breathe – it is unsurprising that obese people get out of breath very easily. In addition, overweight and obese people have greater amounts of fat tissue deposited around the upper airway, particularly the larynx. This may impair the flow of air through these passages during sleep. Changes to the respiratory function are most troublesome during sleep, with subjects (or their partners) complaining of loud snoring and experiencing restlessness. These are the symptoms of obstructive sleep apnoea (temporary cessation of breathing), which is a serious and potentially disabling condition.

Research evidence 9: sleep apnoea

In the Swedish Obese Study,[33] which examined over 3,000 subjects with a BMI above 35, 50% of the men and one-third of the women reported snoring and apnoea. In contrast, only 15.5% of Swedish men of comparable age but normal BMI were self-reported snorers. Several studies have shown an increased risk of myocardial infarction (heart attack) and cerebral infarction (stroke) in sleep apnoea.

Reproductive function

2.23   The association between obesity and abnormalities of reproductive function is well recognised; decreased libido and impotence are common in extremely overweight men, and there is a greater incidence of altered menstrual periods, infertility and complications of pregnancy in obese women.[34] In over-weight and obese subjects, weight loss frequently reverses the changes and restores a normal menstrual cycle and fertility to women.

Liver function

2.24   Obesity may be associated with alterations in liver function that result from the accumulation of fat in the liver. This is known as non-alcoholic steatohepatitis (NASH) and may predispose to the later development of cirrhosis. NASH is often first seen in children.

2.25   Alcohol consumption will accentuate the damage caused to the liver
by fat in overweight subjects and is therefore likely to accelerate liver fibrosis
and cirrhosis. Hence there is a double jeopardy between two important
modern lifestyle diseases – obesity and alcohol misuse.

Research evidence 10: liver function

Forty per cent of patients with NASH are overweight or obese, 20% have type 2
diabetes and 20% are hyperlipidaemic.[35] Tissue evidence of fibrosis and/or cirrhosis
is seen in up to 50% of patients. Most patients who initially show fibrosis, develop
cirrhosis after 10 years.

Gallstones

2.26   Gall bladder disease is a well-recognised complication of obesity in men
and women. Increasing BMI is associated with a substantially increased risk of
the development of gallstones: the risk for women with a BMI over 45 is seven-
fold higher than for women with normal weight.[36] The risk of gallstone
formation increases in the obese during rapid weight loss[37] and this underlines
the reason for caution in the use of 'crash diets'.

Cancer

2.27   Certain forms of cancer are more common in obese people, in particular colorectal and prostate cancer in obese men, and carcinoma of the gall
bladder, breast and endometrium in obese women. It has been estimated that
obesity and overweight are implicated in the development of 10% of colonic
cancers and over 30% of endometrial cancers.[38]

Research evidence 11: cancer

Calculations from a prospective study of more than 900,000 US adult men and
women suggest that deaths from cancer in the USA could be attributable to
overweight and obesity in 14% of men and 20% of women. In subjects with a BMI of
at least 40, death rates from cancer increased by 52% in men and by 62% in women.
In both men and women, increasing BMI was also associated with higher death rates
from cancer of the oesophagus, colon, rectum, liver, gall bladder, pancreas and
kidney. A similar pattern was seen for death due to non-Hodgkin's lymphoma and
myeloma. Significant trends of increasing risk with higher BMI values were observed
for death from cancers of the stomach and prostate in men and for death from
cancers of the breast, uterus, cervix and ovary in women.[39]

Osteoarthritis

2.28   Obesity is a recognised risk factor for the development of osteo-arthritis (OA) because of increased pressure placed on the joints through excess body weight.

2.29   Osteoarthritis is the most prevalent joint disorder of an elderly population. The increased risk of disability attributable to OA alone is as great as that due to heart disease and greater than that due to any other medical disorder in the elderly.[40,41]

Other medical complications and conditions

2.30   Obesity is often associated with other medical complications. These include gastro-oesophageal reflux secondary to a hiatus hernia, lower limb swelling, varicose veins, and excessive sweating.

2.31   As in children, the negative stigma associated with overweight and obesity may contribute to low self-esteem and depression in adults. An increased frequency of psychological and psychiatric problems has been reported in obese adult patients.[42]

Financial costs and economic consequences

2.32   Overweight and obesity, and their associated health consequences, result in a huge financial burden for government, the NHS and society as a whole. The CMO for England has estimated that a general practice with 10,000 patients and five doctors will have to cope with 80 new obese patients each year based on current trends of increasing prevalence, and acknowledges the significant increase in NHS costs.[11] The National Audit Office (NAO) has estimated the costs to the NHS to be at least £0.5 billion a year in terms of treatment, and possibly in excess of £2 billion to the wider economy.[2] The overall annual cost of obesity in the USA has been estimated as $75 billion,[43] and for Australia $1.3 billion,[44] but this is increasing rapidly.

2.33   All of these costs relate to the present generation of adults and take no account of the impact of the rapidly rising prevalence of obesity in children and young people (see Paras 2.2–2.5). There are immeasurable effects on young people that may affect later employment, earnings and social prospects as well as physical and mental healthcare needs.

2.34   The immediate concern is that every generation with an increasing proportion of overweight and obese individuals is storing up severe social, health and economic problems that will be realised in succeeding years, and repeated in future generations.

References

1   World Health Organization. *Diet, nutrition and the prevention of chronic diseases.* Report of a joint WHO/FAO consultation. Geneva: WHO, 2003.

2   National Audit Office. *Tackling obesity in England.* Report by the Comptroller and Auditor General. Norwich: The Stationery Office, 2001. www.nao.gov.uk/guidance/chiefexec2b.htm

3   WHO expert consultation. Appropriate body-mass index for Asian populations and its implications for policy and intervention strategies. *Lancet* 2004;**363**:157–63.

4   Joint Health Surveys Unit (on behalf of the Department of Health). *Health Survey for England, 2002.* Norwich: The Stationery Office, 2003. www.doh.gov.uk/stats/trends1.htm

5   Bundred P, Kitchener D, Buchan I. Prevalence of overweight and obese children between 1989 and 1998: population based series of cross sectional studies. *BMJ* 2001;**322**(7282):326–8.

6   Joint Health Surveys Unit (on behalf of the Department of Health). *Health Survey for England, 2000.* London: The Stationery Office, 2001.

7   Department of Health. *The health of the nation: A strategy for health in England.* London: HMSO, 1992.

8   Whitaker RC, Wright JA, Pepe MS, Seidel KD, Dietz WH. Predicting obesity in young adulthood from childhood and parental obesity (Comment). *N Engl J Med* 1997;**337**(13):869–73.

9   Lobstein TJ, James WP, Cole TJ. Increasing levels of excess weight among children in England. *Int J Obes Relat Metab Disord* 2003;**27**(9):1136–8.

10 Office of Population Censuses and Surveys. OPCS Monitor, ref SS 81/1. London: OPCS, 1981.

11 Department of Health. *Annual Report of the Chief Medical Officer 2002.* London: DH, 2002. www.doh.gov.uk/cmo/annualreport2002

12 Barker DJP. *Mothers, babies and health in later life.* Edinburgh: Churchill Livingstone, 1998.

13 Kopelman PG. Obesity as a medical problem. *Nature* 2000;**404**:635–43.

14 Hubert HB, Feinleib M, McNamara PM, Castelli WP. Obesity as an independent risk factor for cardiovascular disease: a 26-year follow-up of participants in the Framingham heart study. *Circulation* 1983;**67**:968–77.

15 Reilly JJ, Methven E, Mc Dowell ZC, Hacking B. Health consequences of obesity. *Arch Dis Child* 2003;**88**:748–52.

16 Ehtisham S, Barrett TG. The emergence of type 2 diabetes in childhood. *Ann Clin Biochem* 2004;**41**:10–16.

17 Dean H, Flett B. Natural history of type 2 diabetes diagnosed in childhood: long term follow-up in young adult years. *Diabetes* 2002;**51**(Suppl 2):A24–A25 (abstract).

18 Calle EE, Thun MJ, Petrelli JM, Rodriguez C *et al.* Body-mass index and mortality in a prospective cohort of US adults. *N Engl J Med* 1999;**341**:1097–105.

19 Stevens J, Cai J, Pamuk ER, Williamson DF *et al.* The effect of age on the association between body-mass index and mortality. *N Engl J Med* 1998;**338**:1–7.

20 Peeters A, Barendregt JJ, Willekens F, Mackenbach JP *et al.* Obesity in adulthood and its consequences for life expectancy: a life-table analysis. *Ann Intern Med* 2003;**138**:24–32.

21 Colditz GA, Willett WC, Rotnitsky A, Manson JE. Weight gain as a risk factor for clinical diabetes in women. *Arch Intern Med* 1995;**122**:481–6.

22 Chan JM, Rimm EB, Colditz GA, Stampfer MJ, Willett WC. Obesity, fat distribution and weight gain as risk factors for clinical diabetes in men. *Diabetes Care* 1994;**17**:961–9.

23 Kenchaiah S, Evans JC, Levy D, Wilson PWF *et al.* Obesity and the risk of heart failure. *N Engl J Med* 2002;**347**:305–13.

24 Willet WC, Manson JE, Stampfer MJ, Colditz GA *et al.* Weight, weight change and coronary heart disease in women. *JAMA* 1995;**273**:461–5.

25 Eriksson P, Reynisdottir S, Lonnqvist F, Stemme V *et al.* Adipose tissue secretion of plasminogen activator-1 in non-obese and obese individuals. *Diabetologia* 1998;**41**:65–71.

26 Kooistra T, Bosma P, Tons H, van den Berg AP *et al.* Plasminogen activator-1: biosynthesis and mRNA levels are increased by insulin in cultured hepatocytes. *Thromb Haemost* 1989;**62**:723–8.

27 Shimomura I, Funahashi T, Takahashi M, Maeda K *et al.* Enhanced expression of PAI-1 in visceral fat: a possible contributor to vascular disease in obesity. *Nature Med* 1996;**7**:800–3.

28 Juhan-Vague I, Pyke SDM, Alessi MC *et al.* Fibrinolytic factors and the risk of myocardial infarction or sudden death in patients with angina pectoris. *Circulation* 1996;**94**:2057–63.

29 Frayn, Williams CM, Arner P. Are increased plasma non-esterified fatty acid concentrations a risk marker for coronary heart disease and other chronic diseases? *Clin Sci* 1996;**90**:243–53.

30 Reaven GM. Banting Lecture 1988. Role of insulin in human disease. *Diabetes* 1988;**37**:1595–607.

31 Lapidus L, Bengtsson C, Larsson B, Pennart K *et al.* Distribution of adipose tissue and risk of cardiovascular disease and death: a 12 year follow up of participants in the population study of women in Gothenburg, Sweden. *BMJ* 1984;**289**:1257–61.

32 Larsson B, Svardsudd K, Welin L, Wilhelmsen l *et al.* Abdominal adipose tissue distribution, obesity and risk of cardiovascular disease and death: 13 year follow up of participants in the study of men born in 1913. *BMJ* 1984;**288**:1401–4.

33 Grunstein RR, Stenlof K, Hedner J, Sjostrom L. Impact of obstructive apnoea and sleepiness on metabolic and cardiovascular risk factors in the Swedish Obese Subjects (SOS) Study. *Int J Obesity* 1995;**19**:410–18.

34 Kopelman PG. Neuroendocrine function in obesity. *Clin Endocrinol* 1988;**28**:675–89.

35 James O, Day C. Non-alcoholic steatohepatitis: another disease of affluence. *Lancet* 1999;**353**:1634–6.

36 Stampfer MJ, Maclure MK, Colditz GA, Manson JE, Willett WC. Risk of symptomatic gallstones in women with severe obesity. *Am J Clin Nutrition* 1992;**55**:652–8.

37 Festi D, Colecchia A, Orsini M, Sangermano A *et al.* Gallbladder motility and gallstone formation in obese patients following very low calorie diets. Use it (fat) to lose it (well). *Int J Obesity* 1998;**22**:592–600.

38 Bergstrom A, Pisani P, Tenet V, Wolk A, Adami HO. Overweight as an avoidable cause of cancer in Europe. *Int J Cancer* 2001;**91**(3):421–30.

39 Calle EE, Rodriguez C, Walker-Thurmond K, Thun MJ. Overweight, obesity and mortality from cancer in a prospectively studied cohort of US adults. *N Engl J Med* 2003;**348**:1625–38.

40 Peat G, McCarney R, Croft P. Knee pain and osteoarthritis in older adults: a review of community burden and current use of health care. *Ann Rheum Dis* 2001;**60**:91–7.

41 Sharma L, Song J, Felson D, Cahue S *et al.* The mechanism of the effect of obesity in knee osteoarthritis. *Arthritis Rheum* 2000;**43**:568–75.

42 Doll HA, Petersen SEK, Stewart-Brown SL. Obesity and physical and emotional well-being: associations between body mass index, chronic illness, and the physical and mental components of the SF-36 questionnaire. *Obesity Res* 2000;**8**:160–70.

43 Editorial. Who pays in the obesity war? *Lancet* 2004;**363**(9406).

44 National Health and Medical Research Council. *Overweight and obesity guidelines.* Australia: NHMRC, 2003. www.nhmrc.gov.au/media/rel2003/obese.htm

3 The causes of obesity: addressing the energy balance

Why is the health balance wrong?

3.1   The World Health Organization (WHO) first highlighted that obesity was the fastest growing threat to health in both developing and developed countries in 1997.[1] Why is the UK population getting fatter? The simple answer is to do with energy balance: people are eating too much for the amount of physical activity they do (Fig 3.1).

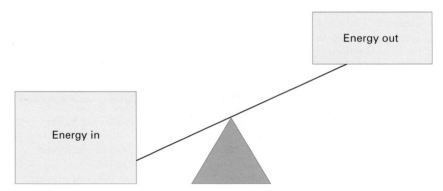

Energy out

Energy in

Fig 3.1 An unhealthy balance: people are taking in too much energy (food) for the energy they expend.

3.2   Energy is needed by the body to maintain body functions, for active movement, and for growth and repair. It is provided by food and drink, and can be measured in calories or joules. The total amount of energy required by individuals depends mainly on their level of physical activity and their body weight. The more active and the heavier they are, the more energy they require.[2]

3.3   A balanced diet and physical activity are both essential to maintaining health, defined by the WHO as: 'Physical, mental and social well-being and not merely the absence of disease or infirmity'.[3] Weight is gained when the body's energy intake exceeds its energy expenditure. It has been estimated that the average adult whose daily energy input is just 60 calories more than their energy output will become obese within 10 years.[4]

3.4   There is an underlying genetic basis to the control of body weight –
some people put on weight more easily than others and this is particularly
apparent in some families (familial tendency). However, the rapid increase in
obesity in the last few years cannot be explained by changes in the gene pool,
but must be caused by environmental and social change.[5]

3.5   This rise in levels of obesity is likely to be due to both an increase in
energy taken in and a decrease in energy expended.

Energy out

3.6   Over the last 10 years, average adult energy expenditure may have
decreased by as much as 30%.[6] In England, only 37% of men and 25% of
women achieve the recommended weekly physical activity level (Box 3.1).[7]
Less than 20% of middle-aged and older adults are sufficiently active for
health.[8]

3.7   Low levels of physical activity are also seen in children:[9] in England,
almost one-third of boys and two-fifths of girls do not achieve the recommended weekly physical activity level (Box 3.1).[10] English schools are at the
bottom of the European league in terms of time allocated to physical education
in primary and secondary schools. Only 5% of children use their bicycles as a
form of transport in the UK, compared to 60–70% in the Netherlands, and
30–40% are now taken to school by car, compared to 9% in 1971.[8]

Box 3.1 Percentages of children and adults achieving recommended weekly physical activity levels in England.[7,10]			
Boys	70%	Men	37%
Girls	61%	Women	25%

Energy in

3.8   The majority of people in the UK do not follow the nutritional
guidelines recommended by health professionals. The recent National Diet
and Nutrition Survey (2002) clearly shows that the nation is eating too much
of the wrong types of food and not enough healthy foods (Box 3.2).[11]

Box 3.2 Diet of children and adults in England.[12]

Overall, adults in England are eating:
▸ more than twice the amount of saturated fat they need
▸ half the fruit and vegetables needed
▸ half the fibre needed
▸ half the fish needed.

Overall, children aged 4 to 18 in England are eating:
▸ more than twice the amount of saturated fat they need
▸ a quarter of the fruit and vegetables needed
▸ more than twice the salt needed
▸ more than twice the sugar needed.

Complex factors that influence obesity levels

3.9   A wide range of economic, environmental, social and cultural factors influence an individual's lifestyle and are likely to have contributed to the 'obesity epidemic'. People do not choose to become fat. Although it is impossible to establish a direct causal link between environmental/cultural factors and the rise in obesity levels, there are obvious associations between changing environments and increasing waistlines, particularly in the following areas:

▸ work and leisure time
▸ town and transport planning
▸ food production and marketing
▸ lifestyle messages
▸ health inequalities.

Work and leisure time

3.10   The way in which work and leisure time is spent has changed at all stages of life, resulting in a major shift in eating and physical activity patterns:

▸ Jobs are more sedentary.
▸ Labour-saving devices, from lifts to remote TV/video controls, have reduced daily activity levels.
▸ Car use has increased and people walk/cycle less.
▸ Screen-based entertainment (TV, computer) has increased significantly.
▸ Less time is spent preparing meals and more processed food is consumed.

▶ Both eating out (11% of energy intake)[13] and snacking/grazing are more common.

▶ Alcohol intake in women and young men has increased[14] (Box 3.3).

Box 3.3 Alcohol consumption.

Alcohol contributes to energy balance, and so changing patterns of alcohol ingestion, particularly in the young, are likely to be important. A pint of beer or a single gin and tonic will each contain about 200 calories. The effects of alcohol on body mass depend on several factors including:

▶ the percentage of daily calories taken as alcohol
▶ the type of alcohol and pattern of drinking
▶ the metabolism of alcohol
▶ the effects of alcohol on appetite
▶ sex and age
▶ whether studies look at population trends (epidemiology) or the responses of individuals in a laboratory (physiology).

Although chronic misusers are usually thinner than average, long-term population studies of non-dependent drinkers suggest both an increase in weight and a redistribution of fat centrally (a higher risk pattern), particularly in men.[15]

Town and transport planning

3.11   In 2000, there were over 24 million cars in the UK. This equates to approximately one car for every two adults.[16] The shift over the last 50 years to private car use has encouraged inactive lifestyles, both by creating an expectation of door-to-door convenience and by making roads less safe for walking and cycling. Town planning in recent years has favoured the car user, and walking is now seen by many as 'the mode of transport for those who have no alternative'.[17] There has been a reduction in local grocery stores and an increase in larger edge-of-town supermarkets, which has left an increasing number of communities and neighbourhoods without easy access to healthy, affordable food.[18] An inequity of access to basic amenities, such as supermarkets, food markets, leisure centres, parks and playgrounds, exists between those with and those without private transport.

Food production

3.12   Diet and nutrition in the UK are strongly influenced by the price and availability of food; European and international policies therefore have a considerable impact on the UK diet. For example, the European Union currently produces an excess of dairy products (including butter), but not enough fruit and vegetables or at sufficiently low prices. At present, the Common Agricultural Policy does not have health improvement as a principal aim.[19]

3.13   The intake of processed foods, which are generally high in sugar and fat, has increased, and much of it is marketed in bigger portions (super-sizing). Food aimed primarily at children tends to be higher in fat and/or sugar than food produced for adults.

Food marketing

3.14   Food marketing and advertising reflect heavy investment and great sophistication, and permeate all levels of society. Ninety per cent of food advertising screened during children's broadcasts is for foods high in fat, salt and/or sugar.[20] A recent review of the effects of food promotion to children, prepared for the Food Standards Agency (FSA), concluded:[21]

▸ Food advertising to children is extensive.
▸ The diet being advertised is less healthy than the recommended diet for children.
▸ Children enjoy and engage with food promotion.
▸ Food promotion is affecting preference, purchase behaviour and consumption.
▸ The effect is independent of other factors and operates at both brand and food category level.

3.15   The food industry argues that advertising affects people's choice of brand, but not their food choices, ie an advert can make people buy one chocolate bar instead of another, but cannot make people decide to buy a chocolate bar as opposed to a piece of fruit. However, the FSA report shows a clear link between the food advertised to children and the type of food they consume.

Lifestyle messages

3.16   Professionals and the public receive, interpret and pass on complex and often contradictory messages about food, diet and physical activity. These come from a variety of sources, such as government, health professionals, schools, food manufacturers, retailers, advertisers, the media, as well as families, friends and colleagues. With such a plethora of information and opinion, it is not surprising that people are confused about what constitutes a healthy lifestyle. Of those interviewed for an FSA consumer survey (2000):

▶ only 12% thought that current food labelling was 'very easy to understand'; overall understanding of fat, sugar and salt levels and ingredient labelling was poor

▶ just over one-third knew what the recommended fruit and vegetable intake was

▶ over 50% did not know how many grams of fat there were in 100 g of a product labelled '80% fat free'.

3.17   The evidence suggests that many people lack quite basic understanding about healthy eating and active living, so there is a need for a sustained campaign, using simple, practical messages, to promote healthy and active living (see Chapter 4).

Health inequalities

3.18   In the developed world, obesity is a health problem that is exacerbated by low socio-economic status. In the UK, people living in households without an earner consume more calories than those living in households with one or more earners. Poorer households eat less fruit and vegetables, salad, wholemeal bread, wholegrain and high-fibre cereals and oily fish, and more white bread, full-fat milk, table sugar and processed meat products. Furthermore, poorer households in poorer communities are less likely to have access to healthy, affordable food and suitable recreational facilities (Box 3.4).

Box 3.4 Main barriers to healthy eating and adequate physical activity for those on a low income.

Barriers to healthy eating
▶ Low income and debt
▶ Inaccessibility of affordable, healthy foods
▶ Lack of facilities/skills/time to cook
▶ Lack of accessible information on nutrition
▶ Poor literacy and numeracy skills, affecting understanding of food labelling and nutritional information

▶

Box 3.4 Main barriers to healthy eating and adequate physical activity for those on a low income. *(continued)*

Barriers to adequate physical activity

▶ Lack of access to affordable sports facilities

▶ Poor urban environments

▶ Lack of community safety

▶ Sedentary lifestyles

▶ Limited encouragement of exercise at school

▶ Limited play facilities

▶ Lack of safe places to play or exercise

Getting the health balance right

3.19   A balanced diet and regular physical activity maintain a healthy weight and have multiple health benefits throughout life. Obesity can be prevented by maintaining the right energy balance – ensuring that energy intake equals energy expenditure (Fig 3.2).

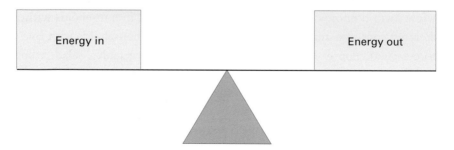

Fig 3.2 A healthy balance: energy intake equals energy expenditure.

3.20   This section describes what a healthy lifestyle consists of, and what individuals need to do to achieve a healthy balance. Chapter 4 will discuss what changes need to be made at national and local level in order to enable individuals to make healthy choices.

Energy out

3.21   Physical activity, defined as 'any bodily movement produced by the muscles that results in energy expenditure'[22] has significant benefits to physical and mental health throughout life.[23] Regular physical activity helps to:[24]

▶ reduce the risk of cardiovascular disease, particularly coronary heart disease (CHD)

▶ prevent or delay the onset of high blood pressure, and control where present

▶ prevent the onset of type 2 diabetes, and improve its control where present

▶ regulate body weight

▶ reduce the risk of osteoporosis

▶ reduce the risk of colon cancer

▶ improve coordination, strength and balance in older people, and hence reduce falls and fractures

▶ reduce symptoms of anxiety and depression

▶ promote participation in a range of activities and networks

▶ increase personal skills, self-esteem and enjoyment.

Box 3.5 Current recommendations on physical activity.

Adults:
A total of at least 30 minutes of moderately intensive activity (eg brisk walking) on at least five days a week[25]

Children:
A total of at least one hour of moderately intensive physical activity every day[26]

3.22   Box 3.5 gives the current recommendations on physical activity levels for adults and children, and Fig 3.3 shows a range of activities equivalent to walking for 30 minutes.

3.23   Active people are slimmer than sedentary people, and even small increases in physical activity can help to control weight. In addition to raising levels of planned physical activity (eg swimming, walking, playing football, an aerobics or dance class), energy output can be increased during daily household and occupational chores. Changes in routine, such as using the stairs rather than the lift, can make a difference and help to maintain or restore energy balance.

Activity	Time (min)
Washing and waxing a car	45–60
Washing windows or floors	45–60
Playing volleyball	45
Playing touch football	30–45
Gardening	30–45
Walking 3 km	40
Basketball (shooting practice)	30
Cycling 8 km	30
Dancing fast	30
Pushing a pushchair for 2.5 km	30
Raking leaves	30
Walking 3.5 km	35
Water aerobics	30
Swimming laps	20
Wheelchair basketball	20
Basketball game	15–20
Cycling 6.5 km	15
Skipping	15
Running	15
Stair walking	15

Less vigorous
More time

More vigorous
Less time

Fig 3.3 Different activities equivalent to walking at a moderate intensity for 30 minutes.[22] (Reproduced with permission from the BHF National Centre for Physical Activity and Health; original figure adapted from *Physical activity and health: a report of the Surgeon General*.)[27]

Energy in

3.24   A balanced diet provides the energy (calories) and nutrients needed, not just to survive, but also to stay fit and healthy. The benefits of a healthy diet begin before conception and continue until old age: a balance in dietary intake across different food groups is essential for health. If weight needs to be lost, a balanced reduction across the different food groups is advisable, rather than a diet that excludes certain food groups entirely.

3.25   There are five food groups (Fig 3.4):

1 bread, other cereals and potatoes
2 fruit and vegetables
3 milk and dairy foods

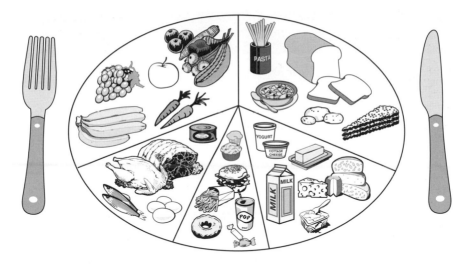

Fig 3.4 The five food groups: fruit and vegetables; bread, other cereals and potatoes; milk and dairy foods; foods containing fat/sugar; meat, fish and protein alternatives. The size of the segments represents the recommended proportions of each group in the diet. (Adapted from *The balance of good health*; reproduced with permission from the Food Standards Agency.)

4   meat, fish and protein alternatives

5   foods containing fat and foods containing sugar.

3.26   The British Nutrition Foundation recently issued guidelines on how to achieve a healthy, balanced diet.[28] People should choose a variety of foods from the first four groups every day, and food from the fifth group should be eaten sparingly. A balanced diet should be based on breads, potatoes and cereals, should be rich in fruit and vegetables, with moderate amounts of milk and dairy products, meat, fish or protein alternatives, and limited amounts of food containing fat or sugar.

Box 3.6 Simple dietary messages for children over five and adults.[12]

▸ Enjoy your food.
▸ Eat at least five portions of fruit and vegetables a day.
▸ Eat starchy food – bread, potatoes, rice and pasta (wholegrain, ie containing fibre).
▸ Increase fibre intake.   ▸

Box 3.6 Simple dietary messages for children over five and adults.[12]
(continued)

▶ Eat fish at least twice a week (one oily).

▶ Eat less fat.

▶ Eat less sugar.

▶ Eat no more than 5 oz red meat per day.

▶ Phase out added salt.

References

1   World Health Organization. *Obesity: preventing and managing the global epidemic.* Geneva: WHO, 1997.
2   British Nutrition Foundation website: www.nutrition.org.uk/information/energy&nutrients/energy.html
3   World Health Organization. *Preamble to the Constitution.* Geneva: WHO, 1948.
4   Lobstein T. Are the calorie counters getting it wrong? *Food magazine* 2003; July/September **62**:19. London: Food Commission.
5   Obesity Resource Information Centre. *Why do people become obese?* Bristol: ORIC, 1997.
6   Obesity Resource Information Centre. *Physical activity and obesity.* Bristol: ORIC, 1997.
7   Joint Health Surveys Unit. *Health Survey for England: cardiovascular disease 1998.* London: The Stationery Office, 1999.
8   Obesity: the biggest unrecognised public health problem? *NW Health Bulletin* March 2002;**2**:4.
9   Reilly JJ, Jackson DM, Montgomery C, Kelly LA *et al.* Total energy expenditure and physical activity in young Scottish children: mixed longitudinal study. *Lancet* 2004;**363**:211–12.
10 Joint Health Surveys Unit (on behalf of the Department of Health). *Health Survey for England: the health of young people 2002.* London: The Stationery Office, 2003.
11 Office for National Statistics/ Medical Research Council Human Nutrition Research. *The National Diet and Nutrition Survey: adults aged 19 to 64 years. Volume 1.* Norwich: The Stationery Office, 2002.
12 Press V. *Nutrition and food poverty.* London: National Heart Forum, Faculty of Public Health (2004, in press).
13 Department for Environment, Food and Rural Affairs/Office for National Statistics. *National Food Survey 2000: annual report on food expenditure, consumption and nutrient intakes.* London: The Stationery Office, 2001.
14 Department of Health. *Annual Report of the Chief Medical Officer 2002.* London: DH, 2002. www.doh.gov.uk/cmo/annualreport2002.
15 Wannamethee SG, Shaper AG. Alcohol, body weight and weight gain in middle-aged men. *Am J Clin Nutr* 2003;**77**(5):1312–7.
16 Sustrans. *Healthy and active travel newssheet,* 2001. www.sustrans.org.uk/downloads/989A75_fh01.pdf
17 House of Commons Select Committee on Environment, Transport and Regional Affairs. Eleventh Report, para 19.
18 Simms A, Oram J, MacGillivray A, Drury J. *Ghost town Britain: the threat from economic globalisation to livelihoods, liberty and local economic freedom.* London: New Economics Foundation, 2002.

19 European Health Forum. *Health at the heart of CAP*. Health and Common Agricultural Policy Reform: Opinion and Proposals of an Expert Working Group. London: Faculty of Public Health, 2002. www.fph.org.uk/publications_press_and_communications/Publications/Publications.shtml

20 Sustain: the Alliance for Better Food and Farming. *TV dinners: what's being served up by the advertisers?* London: Sustain, 2001:v.

21 Hastings G, Stead M, McDermott L, Forsyth A *et al* (prepared on behalf of the Food Standards Agency). *Review of research on the effects of food promotion to children*. London: FSA, 2003.

22 National Centre for Physical Activity and Health. *A physically active lifestyle information pack*. www.bhfactive.org.uk/resources/active_lifestyle.doc

23 Kesaniemi YA, Danforth E, Jensen MD, Kopelman PG *et al*. Dose-response issues concerning physical activity and health: an evidence-based symposium. *Sports Exercise* 2001;**33**(suppl):S351-8.

24 Faculty of Public Health and National Heart Forum. *Let's get moving! A physical activity handbook for developing local programmes*. London: Faculty of Public Health, 2001.

25 Department of Health. *Strategy statement on physical activity*. London: DH, 1996.

26 Cavill N, Biddle S, Sallis JF. Health-enhancing physical activity for young people: Statement of the United Kingdom Expert Consensus Conference. *Pediatr Exercise Sci* 2001;**31**:12–25.

27 US Department of Health and Human Services. *Physical activity and health: a report of the Surgeon General*. Atlanta: US Department of Health and Human Services, Centers for Disease Control and Prevention, and National Center for Chronic Disease Prevention and Health Promotion.

28 British Nutrition Foundation. *Healthy eating: a whole diet approach*. London: BNF, 2003.

4 Strategies to prevent obesity

Principles

The challenge

4.1 To prevent obesity, the nation has to consume less energy and be more physically active. Most people, especially those prone to overweight, are well aware of these basic principles but, for various reasons, find it difficult to follow them. The challenge, in tipping the balance towards a trimmer and slimmer nation, is to help people overcome the many barriers to a healthier lifestyle.

Tipping the balance – 'the three E's'

4.2 As with any collective behaviour change, success is most likely if progress is made on three broad fronts – environment, empowerment and encouragement (Fig 4.1).

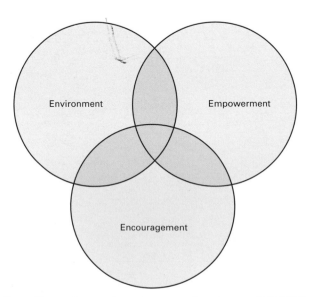

Fig 4.1 The three E's: environment, empowerment and encouragement.

Environment – creating an environment (physical, social and economic) which predisposes to healthy eating and active living. The purpose is to make the healthier choices the easier choices by removing barriers such as high cost or difficult access. This includes tackling inequities caused by exclusion, disadvantage or poverty.

Examples:

▶ Free fruit in schools

▶ Healthy school policies, eg healthy catering, fruit tuckshops, plentiful drinking water, breakfast clubs, after-school activities (including dance), and an absence of vending machines dispensing sugary drinks and fatty, sugary or salty snacks

▶ Conveniently placed food outlets offering healthier choices at affordable prices, including food 'co-ops' in which community groups purchase foods direct from growers or wholesale suppliers and sell at cost to people on low incomes

▶ Agricultural policies and food subsidies that help to provide healthier choices at affordable prices

▶ Safe walking and cycling routes to school and work

▶ Town planning that discourages car use

▶ Safe, accessible parks

▶ Buildings designed to encourage stair use and discourage lift/escalator use

▶ Bike racks and shower facilities in workplaces

▶ Cheaper and easier access to leisure and sports facilities

▶ Culturally sensitive exercise facilities (eg women-only swimming sessions)

▶ Media-created ethos that a healthy active lifestyle is 'cool'.

Empowerment – giving people, particularly children and young people, knowledge and understanding of the benefits of healthy eating, active living and avoiding overweight, and the life skills to adopt healthy behaviours; boosting confidence and self-esteem, individually and collectively. This includes educating key opinion formers such as health professionals, schoolteachers and the media.

Examples:

▶ Personal, social and health education (PSHE) work in schools

▶ Teaching the principles of healthy eating and cooking skills

▶ Physical education (PE), sports and other supervised physical activities in schools

▶ Teaching citizenship and advocacy skills

▶ Working with communities (eg minority ethnic groups or housing estate residents) to understand their needs for a healthier diet and more exercise, and to demand better access to fresh fruit and vegetables, a leisure centre etc

▶ Health visitors working with new mothers and young families to support and encourage breastfeeding, healthy eating and healthy active play

▶ Nutrition and physical activity and behaviour change modules built into the core basic training of health professionals

▶ Clear messages about healthy eating and physical activity for all age groups.

Encouragement – motivating and prompting people to make the necessary changes to their lifestyles here and now; and triggering action.

Examples:

▶ Active play for pre-school children

▶ Sports and games in schools

▶ Media campaigns (eg the Department of Health's 'Five-a-Day' campaign to promote the consumption of fruit and vegetables; the Health Education Authority's 'Active for Life' campaign to promote a more active everyday lifestyle)

▶ Trigger messages (eg low fat/sugar logos on packaged foods; low calorie options on menus; walk prompts on lifts and escalators)

▶ Healthy walks groups

▶ Sports clubs

▶ Fun-runs, aerobathons, and other mass activities

▶ Life insurance health checks

▶ Motivational counselling in primary care

▶ Incentives/rewards for 'active transport' (eg walking, cycling, etc) to school or work.

All three basic elements are essential and interdependent.

Target groups

4.3   Although everyone needs to watch their weight, the national pro-gramme to tackle obesity is likely to be more effective if initiatives are targeted at those individuals, families and communities most prone to overweight, or for whom being overweight poses a higher risk to health. National and local initiatives should therefore target the following three priority groups, with particular attention to individuals, families and communities who may be disadvantaged in terms of age, gender, income, language, culture, ethnicity, ability/disability, or geographical location:

All children and young people: healthy eating and an active lifestyle should be promoted to prevent the onset of overweight and to develop healthy habits for life.

Children and young people who are overweight or obese: weight control should be promoted and the risks associated with overweight and obesity reduced. Priority should be given to those for whom obesity would confer extra risk of ill health (eg children with diabetes, or musculoskeletal problems), and to those suffering adverse consequences (eg bullying and low self-esteem).

Adults with a tendency to become overweight or obese: weight control should be promoted and the risks associated with overweight and obesity reduced. Priority should be given to those at particular risk of obesity (eg through a family predisposition, people giving up smoking, pregnant women), or for whom obesity would confer extra risk of ill health (eg people with high blood pressure, diabetes, depression, musculoskeletal problems).

Prevention of obesity at national level

4.4 There is evidence from around the world that centrally coordinated, multi-agency, strategic approaches to tackling obesity are more likely to achieve substantial and sustained results.[1] Such approaches are often contained within broader health improvement strategies.

4.5 All four UK countries already have national health improvement strategies in place which encompass the promotion of healthy eating and an active lifestyle. In England, the Government White Paper on health improvement, *Saving lives: our healthier nation* (1999),[2] sets targets for reducing the impact of such major killers as coronary heart disease (CHD), strokes and cancers. *Saving lives* proposes action at three levels: individual, community and government (national).

4.6   All four UK countries also have more disease-focused plans to prevent and treat the major diseases such as CHD, stroke, diabetes and cancers. In England, for example, there are national service frameworks (NSFs) to tackle cancers, mental health, CHD, diabetes, health problems in older people (including stroke and falls), and children's health. Each of these will have a major impact on overweight/obesity in various ways, and the CHD NSF specifies reducing obesity as a designated priority with stated objectives and milestones.[3]

4.7   All four UK countries have specific plans to improve the national diet or increase physical activity and sport. For example, Scotland has its diet action plan, *Eating for health*,[4] and its physical activity strategy, *Let's make Scotland more active*,[5] Wales has its *Food and well being*[6] and *Healthy and active lifestyles in Wales: a framework for action*,[7] England has its *Game plan*[8] and forthcoming physical activity strategy and food and health action plan, and in Northern Ireland healthy eating and physical activity strategies are incorporated into *Investing for health*.[9] The UK-wide Food Standards Agency (FSA) is doing much to promote healthy eating by encouraging the food industry to improve the nutritional quality of processed and convenience foods, to promote healthier alternatives and to develop simple nutritional labelling.

4.8   As shown in Chapter 3, obesity and health are closely linked to socio-economic status. All four UK countries have cross-government programmes to reduce the socio-economic divide and tackle health inequalities. In England, for example, the Government has published *Tackling health inequalities: a programme for action* which focuses on the wider determinants of health[10] (Fig 4.2). Many national initiatives are linked to this: for example, reform of the Welfare Food Scheme to ensure that 800,000 children, pregnant women and mothers from low-income families have a healthy diet; and the New Opportunities Fund programme to develop and improve sports facilities for around 2,300 schools and raise standards of physical education, especially in disadvantaged areas.

4.9   As well as these health improvement strategies, all four UK countries have developed a plethora of strategies related to other socio-economic and infrastructure issues which, although not primarily intended to have an impact on health, nevertheless will do so in a multiplicity of ways. Many of these will directly or indirectly affect people's dietary and exercise patterns. Examples include strategies/policies in the following areas:

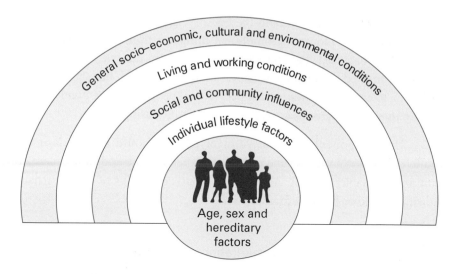

Fig 4.2 The wider determinants of health.[11]

- transport
- agriculture and food production
- environment and housing
- education
- employment
- crime and community safety
- welfare and benefits
- social care.

4.10   To succeed in tackling the time-bomb of obesity, each country in the UK needs a cross-governmental, 'joined-up', high-level strategy which gathers together all these elements and welds them into a coherent, whole-system approach to the prevention and treatment of overweight and obesity.

Public education and social marketing

4.11   In the developed world, there are a number of national public education campaigns that have succeeded in raising awareness of the issues and promoting healthier eating and more active living, the most notable example being Finland's North Karelia Project.[12] Multimedia public education approaches have proved effective in reducing weight gain in two large-scale community-based programmes in the USA.[13,14] As part of its strategy, central government should mount a promotional campaign to motivate the public to eat a healthy, balanced diet and adopt a more active lifestyle. The campaign should be directed at everyone, whatever their background, but should particularly aim to engage children, young people, and people who are disadvantaged or from those ethnic groups at greatest risk from increasing fatness.

4.12   The component aimed at younger people should use humour and youth 'champions' to convey the message that being active and eating plenty of fruit and vegetables is 'cool'. All the social marketing skills of the advertising industry should be brought to bear.

Food and drink production, marketing and retailing

4.13   People's choice of food and drink depends greatly on such factors as price and availability, as well as flavour, quality, convenience and nutritional value. The food industry, from farm gate to consumer's plate, has a key role to play in determining what foods are consumed and in what quantity or balance. The dominant force in this chain is likely to be the supermarkets, which can strongly influence primary producers as well as consumers.

4.14   Ideally, consumers should be presented with a wide choice of foods from which they can select a healthy balance for the family table *at prices the poorest can afford*. Theoretically, the contents of the family shopping trolley should correspond to nationally recommended dietary intakes.[15]

4.15   Much work is currently being undertaken in partnership with the food industry to try to shift consumer demand away from high fat, high sugar, high-calorie products, towards healthier alternatives. However, greater effort is needed to achieve a healthier national diet and, in particular, to increase consumption of fresh fruit and vegetables. This should go beyond simply engaging the food industry in initiatives, and should instead aim for joint working towards good practice as part of the food and advertising industries' corporate social responsibility.

Nutritional labelling

4.16   As people become more aware of the health consequences of what they eat and drink, so it becomes increasingly important for them to have useful nutritional information about each food item. This should include guidance on calorie content. However, it is essential that this is given in an easily understandable form, such as simple symbols indicating 'high', 'medium' and 'low' calorie content. As far as possible, this should be in accordance with the latest European Union nutritional labelling proposals. The Food Standards Agency is leading on this work for the UK.

Promoting 'active transport'

4.17   The national strategy must contain a strong element promoting 'active transport', ie discouraging the unnecessary use of cars, and encouraging walking and cycling. This might involve initiatives regarding town planning, building specifications, road taxation, VAT on bikes, etc. Safety of walkers and cyclists is a key issue. The need for policies which promote and support active transport is recognised by all four UK governments.

Promoting leisure-time physical activity and sport

4.18   Much is already being done to promote leisure-time physical activity and sport. All four UK countries have well-funded non-governmental organisations (NGOs) which promote such sport and leisure activities. All four have comprehensive strategies in place, with clearly identified priority target groups. However, there is still much to be done, particularly in terms of joining up with local strategic partnerships for health and well-being. A key gap is the lack of strong and effective links between the leisure and health sectors.

Promoting healthy schools

4.19   There is evidence to support a multifaceted approach to promoting healthy eating and physical activity in the schools setting, including: curricular and non-curricular education; healthy food and drink choices in school meals, tuckshops and vending machines; and sport, active pursuits and active travel to and from school.[16] For many years, school catering suffered from inadequate budgets and an absence of statutory nutritional standards. In 2001, national nutritional standards were re-introduced and catering budgets were made the responsibility of school governors. Hopefully, these changes will result in healthier choices for all schoolchildren. In particular, there should always be an attractive choice of fresh fruit on offer in school dining rooms.

4.20   In England, the National School Fruit Scheme, offering every child in England aged four to six a free piece of fruit each school day, has been successfully piloted and will be fully operational nationwide from 2004. The Government has also recently launched its 'Food in schools' programme, jointly run by the Department of Health and Department for Education and Skills, which will involve over 500 schools in eight pilot projects around the country, looking at a range of initiatives from breakfast clubs and lunchboxes to healthier vending machines, fruit tuckshops, and after-school cookery classes.

4.21   Pressure on the school curriculum has been blamed for the gradual erosion of teaching time devoted to sports, active games and physical education. There has also been a trend toward selling off school playing fields in order to help balance hard-pressed education budgets. These issues are being actively addressed and the trends reversed. There is now a minimum standard of two hours of moderate physical activity in school time per week. Very large capital sums, from such sources as the New Opportunities Fund, are being invested in schools' sport and physical education facilities and equipment, focusing on the more deprived areas of the country.

4.22   In England, the National Healthy School Standard[17] aims to encourage schools to develop a 'whole school' approach to health and to consider diet and physical activity (along with sex and relationships, drugs and alcohol, tobacco and citizenship) in all aspects of school life. It is part of the Healthy Schools Programme, led jointly by the Department for Education and Skills and the Department of Health. Similar initiatives exist in other UK countries. However, it is up to the individual school to decide its Healthy School priorities, and in many cases education in sex and relationships, drugs and alcohol takes precedence over attention to diet and physical activity.

4.23   One aspect of the whole school approach is to ensure that healthy eating messages are consistent across the classroom, dining room, tuckshop and vending machine. The tuckshop and vending machine, in particular, should not promote sugary or fatty snacks or sugared drinks. School governors should consider banning these items from the tuckshop or vending machine. At the same time, they should ensure the easy availability of plain drinking water. In Scotland, the provision of water and fruit juice in school vending machines is now mandatory and advertisements on the front of the machines promoting sugar-sweetened drinks and fatty or sugary snacks are banned.

4.24   It is important that these school-based initiatives are sustained and built upon, involving parents and local communities.

NHS priorities, planning and performance

4.25   Recent NHS priorities and planning guidance[18] continues to focus on health services and pays scant attention to tackling obesity or promoting healthy eating and active living. Any references to these aspects tend to be inferred in longer-term targets concerning CHD and cancer, with an emphasis on adults. The urgency of the problem among children and young people is barely acknowledged. It is most important that the prevention and management of overweight and obesity, prioritising children and young people, be given greater prominence in future priority-setting and planning for the NHS and social care.

4.26   With regard to adults, an important opportunity now exists with the implementation of the new General Medical Services (GMS) contract. The contract's Quality and Outcomes Framework is designed to raise organisational and clinical standards in primary care, with an emphasis on team-working and nurse-led chronic disease management. Within it is a requirement to record accurate data in a standardised electronic format. This should greatly improve risk management of CHD, stroke, hypertension and diabetes, including the risks associated with overweight and obesity. Along with other initiatives such as the Expert Patients Programme and the Electronic Patient Record, this is expected to contribute greatly to an improved service for managing overweight/obesity, and for monitoring the implementation and effectiveness of programmes to prevent and treat obesity.

4.27   However, there remains a lack of coordination in terms of workforce planning. As more and more overweight patients are assessed as being at risk of cardiovascular disease or diabetes, so this will put a greater strain on local community dietitians and exercise referral services. It is essential that workforce planners factor these trends into their calculations, and provide for extra community dietitians and physical activity coordinators as necessary.

4.28   All NHS trusts should ensure that the management of overweight and obesity is integrated into all relevant clinical programmes.

Research and development

4.29   A comprehensive, national R&D programme designed to evaluate methods of achieving sustainable behaviour change in individuals and the community with regard to healthy eating and physical activity is urgently required.

4.30   In particular, there should be increased investment in research into the psychology, sociology and social anthropology of food and drink choice and leisure activities of children and young people – and ways of influencing these behaviours through more effective social marketing of healthier lifestyles. Particular attention needs to be paid to specific ethnic, socio-economic or vulnerable groups.

4.31   There is also a dearth of studies on the cost-effectiveness of interventions on an individual, group or wider community basis.

4.32   More research is required into the role of the physical and economic environment in shaping people's dietary and physical activity choices. Reviews of the impact of the many national and local strategies and policies that influence a population's diet, physical activity patterns and obesity levels need to be conducted.

Prevention programmes at local level

4.33   Sustained change can only be brought about by working in a 'whole system' way across the various sectors locally. Local strategic partnerships (or local community planning partnerships or equivalent) should be urged to develop local action plans to tackle obesity as a priority within their community strategy to promote well-being in their population. In England, a requirement along these lines is included in the Coronary Heart Disease NSF.[3] The Faculty of Public Health has published a toolkit to help local teams develop and implement action plans to tackle obesity.[19]

Potential partners

4.34   Action to prevent obesity at local level will require a coordinated approach involving a range of partner organisations, notably:

▶ community services, such as health visiting and community child health services, eg school nursing

- schools and local education authorities
- leisure services
- local authority planning departments and parks departments
- police and community safety partnerships
- primary care organisations and general practices
- hospitals and community health services
- community groups and voluntary bodies
- local food retailers and caterers
- local employers
- local media.

4.35   Each partner organisation should designate a senior named individual to join a multi-agency steering group to develop and champion the local action plan and oversee its implementation.

Settings approach

4.36   A practical framework for local programmes could be that offered by the so-called 'healthy settings' approach,[20] which focuses interventions in a number of key settings to develop a coordinated programme for obesity prevention. There are many possible settings to develop: from home to hospital, from park to prison, and from community group to club or pub. Each provides a particular opportunity to influence people's eating, drinking and physical activity habits. A simple range of settings for preventing obesity might include:

- home and pre-school
- school
- workplace
- community group
- leisure facility
- retail outlet
- media
- GP surgery, health centre or clinic
- wider population.

4.37 For each setting, various objectives and initiatives should be agreed by the partnership, taking into account the strength of the evidence base. A comprehensive review of the evidence concerning prevention and management of obesity and overweight in children, adolescents and adults has recently been published by the Health Development Agency.[21]

Examples of local initiatives

4.38 Using this approach, Table 4.1 sets out examples of initiatives/actions which could form the components of a local prevention programme.

4.39 Such local programmes should have clear aims and objectives, measurable milestones, and clearly designated roles and responsibilities. Evaluation should be built in from the outset.

Table 4.1 Examples of objectives and initiatives/actions which could be used in a local obesity prevention programme.

Home (preschool)
(Evidence base reviewed by the Centre for Review and Dissemination)[16]

Objective	Initiatives/actions
Promotion of breastfeeding; healthy infant feeding; healthy eating and active lifestyles for young families; 'positive parenting'	▶ Action to promote breastfeeding, appropriate weaning and infant feeding: • One-to-one verbal advice by health visitors or lay workers ('mother-to-mother' schemes) • Breastfeeding 'drop-ins' and 'cafes' • Written support materials • Mass media features • Sure Start programmes • National Breastfeeding Awareness Week
-	▶ Action to promote healthy eating and active living for young children: • 'Positive parenting' advice/classes • Training for childminders and playgroup leaders around healthy eating and active play • Safe play areas

School
(Evidence base reviewed by the Centre for Review and Dissemination)[16]

Objective	Initiatives/actions
A whole-school health-promoting environment	▶ National Healthy Schools Standard ▶ Healthy Schools Partnerships

continued

Teaching healthy eating and cooking skills	▶	Slots for nutrition in the curriculum
	▶	Slots for teaching healthy cooking skills
Healthy school meals, snacks and drinking water	▶	Guidelines on minimum nutritional standards for school meals
	▶	School nutrition policy
	▶	Replacement of sugared drinks and high-calorie snacks (eg in vending machines) with healthier alternatives (eg fruit tuckshops)
	▶	Healthy catering guidelines written into catering contract
	▶	Breakfast clubs
	▶	Drinking water provision
Increased uptake of physical activity and sports	▶	Enjoyable activities, physical education and sports sessions built into the curriculum and after school, including such non-traditional forms as dance in order to develop skills in enjoyable ways
	▶	Safe routes to schools
	▶	'Walking buses' (children walking in supervised groups) and other forms of active travel to/from school
Provision of personalised support and a range of options for children and young people seeking help to control their weight	▶	School nursing service able to support children and parents, and refer on to relevant community and specialist services when needed

Workplace
(Evidence base reviewed by Hennrikus and Jeffery[22] and Shephard)[23]

Objective		Initiatives/actions
Healthy lifestyles amongst staff, including weight control, through healthy eating and increased physical activity	▶	Healthy catering
	▶	Cycle parking racks
	▶	Shower facilities
	▶	Fitness sessions
	▶	Recreational facilities
	▶	Occupational health checks
	▶	Workplace health programmes

Community group

Objective		Initiatives/actions
Healthy eating and physical activity for at-risk groups	▶	Culturally sensitive exercise programmes, eg closed-door, women-only swimming and gym sessions; traditional oriental dance sessions
	▶	Culturally sensitive cooking skills sessions

continued

Leisure facility

Objective		Initiatives/actions
Free or inexpensive access to a wide range of activities	▶	Use of subsidised access schemes for less wealthy local residents
Healthy catering at all leisure venues	▶	Inexpensive healthy choices in leisure centre cafes
	▶	Removal of promotion of less healthy foods and drinks in leisure centres
Coordinated outreach physical activities for specific groups	▶	Healthy walks schemes
	▶	Exercise sessions for older people in care homes
More users walking or cycling to the leisure venue	▶	Cycle parking racks at all leisure venues
Closer links with local schools	▶	Collaboration with local schools to integrate sports and physical activity into curricula and after-school initiatives

Retail outlet

Objective		Initiatives/actions
To harness the power of the retail industry to create a climate where physical activity and healthy eating are considered 'cool'	▶	Engaging large chain stores and other local retailers in promotions and campaigns to sell the 'get fizzical' message to young people
	▶	Involving retailers of fruit and vegetables, juices, etc in the same way

Media

Objective		Initiatives/actions
To harness the power of the local media to create a climate where physical activity and healthy eating are considered 'cool'	▶	Articles/features/interviews in local newspapers and radio/TV programmes
	▶	Promotion of local health days, mini-marathons, healthy cook-ins, aerobathons, and other events
	▶	Agreements preventing children from exposure to unnecessary marketing of high fat/sugar foods and drinks

GP surgery, health centre or clinic
(Evidence base reviewed by Harvey et al)[24]

Objective		Initiatives/actions
Advice and support on healthy eating and physical activity aimed at priority groups	▶	Agreed protocols for providing appropriate advice and support for different types of patient/client
Advice and support for overweight/obese children and young people and their families	▶	Support for all parents in providing a healthy diet and physical activity for and with their children
	▶	Use of existing guidance to support children who wish to control their weight gain, referring for specialist help when needed

continued

Systematic advice and support in managing cases of overweight/obesity	▶	Agreed protocols for managing overweight/obese people using a chronic disease template
Referral of appropriate cases for more specialist advice and support	▶	Agreed criteria for referral to a community dietitian (dietary referral service)
	▶	Agreed criteria for referral to an exercise coordinator/instructor (exercise referral service)
	▶	Agreed criteria for referral to a hospital specialist when needed

Wider population

(There is inconclusive evidence regarding the effectiveness of population-based approaches to promoting healthy eating and physical activity.[21] However, a lack of evidence does not necessarily mean a lack of effectiveness. Rigorous (eg controlled) studies of community-based interventions may be difficult, if not impossible, to undertake, and a pragmatic approach should be adopted, using a range of complementary interventions.)

Objective		*Initiatives/actions*
Healthy eating campaigns	▶	Media campaigns
	▶	Work with local supermarkets
	▶	Healthy eating accreditation schemes for restaurants and food outlets
	▶	Removal of promotion of high fat/sugar foods and drinks from leisure centres, schools, hospitals
Strategies to minimise barriers to healthy eating by improving availability and access	▶	Mapping of 'food deserts'
	▶	Supermarket pricing policies to encourage healthier choices
	▶	Town planning to site food shops selling fruit and vegetables close to areas of deprivation
Group work on healthy eating for higher risk or disadvantaged groups	▶	Identification and mapping of groups at risk
	▶	Culturally sensitive group work
	▶	Peer education
Physical activity and fitness campaigns	▶	Physical activity for older people
	▶	Home-based exercise
	▶	At-risk groups targeted
Increased use of leisure facilities	▶	Improved leisure facilities at affordable prices
Increased walking or cycling to school or workplace	▶	Safe routes to school and workplace
	▶	'Walking buses' (supervised groups of schoolchildren walking to and from school)
Local transport policies which encourage walking and cycling	▶	Provision of reliable, comfortable, frequent, safe and affordable public transport
	▶	Restriction of use of cars in urban areas
	▶	Better traffic calming
	▶	Creation of safe cycling and walking routes
	▶	Wider use of CCTV cameras
Local planning to encourage physical activity	▶	More parks and open spaces
	▶	Better street lighting and safe, clean environments

4.40   Box 4.1 provides a checklist for a local action plan.

Sustained investment

4.41   There are many examples of successful local initiatives that have been funded through time-limited funding sources (eg Neighbourhood Renewal programmes). Unfortunately, some of these initiatives have foundered because of lack of funding. Long-term benefits can only be achieved from sustained financial investment and this should be ensured by giving successful initiatives mainstream funding.

Box 4.1 Checklist for a local action plan.

▸ Make the issue of overweight and obesity a priority for joint action.

▸ Ensure that the plan links with other relevant programmes, for example:
  – health sector programmes such as those promoting child health, healthy adult lifestyles, or healthy old age; and those tackling heart disease, diabetes, stroke, cancer, mental ill-health, and accidents
  – programmes in other sectors such as transport, leisure, education, employment, community safety, housing, etc.

▸ Include elements which help to:
  – create an environment conducive to healthy eating and active living
  – empower individuals, families and communities to make healthier choices
  – encourage individuals, families and communities to make changes now.

▸ Have clear aims and objectives, identify priority target groups, and focus on interventions that have the strongest evidence base.

▸ Include longer-term preventive elements as well as shorter-term obesity management elements.

▸ Include elements which promote healthy eating and an active lifestyle in a variety of settings – healthcare and non-healthcare.

▸ Include health impact assessments of major policy changes in non-healthcare settings.

▸ Include an agreed process for evaluation and performance assessment, including clinical governance of healthcare interventions.

▸ Ensure that the plan is properly resourced and provided with an appropriate infrastructure in terms of staffing, training, premises, equipment, information technology, etc. Local NHS workforce planners should ensure that the likely increased demand for lifestyle counsellors, community dietitians and exercise coordinators is taken into account.

References

1   World Health Organization. *Obesity: preventing and managing the global epidemic. Report of a WHO consultation.* WHO Technical Report Series No 894. Geneva: WHO, 2000.

2 Department of Health. *Saving lives: our healthier nation.* London: DH, 1999.

3 Department of Health. *National Service Framework for Coronary Heart Disease.* London: DH, 2000.

4 Scottish Diet Action Group. *Eating for health: a diet action plan for Scotland.* Edinburgh: Scottish Office, 1996.

5 Physical Activity Task Force. *Let's make Scotland more active: a strategy for physical activity.* Edinburgh: Scottish Executive, 2003.

6 Food Standards Agency Wales and Welsh Assembly Government. *Food and well being: reducing inequalities through a nutrition strategy for Wales.* Cardiff: Welsh Assembly Government, 2003.

7 Office of the Chief Medical Officer. *Healthy and active lifestyles in Wales: a framework for action.* Cardiff: Welsh Assembly Government, 2003.

8 Strategy Unit. *Game plan: a strategy for delivering Government's sport and physical activity objectives.* London: Cabinet Office, 2002.

9 Department of Health, Social Services and Public Safety. *Investing for health.* Belfast: DHSSPS, 2002.

10 Department of Health. *Tackling health inequalities: a programme for action.* London: DH, 2003.

11 Dahlgren G, Whitehead M. *Policies and strategies to promote social equity in health.* Stockholm: Institute for Futures Studies, 1991.

12 Puska P, Tuomilehto J, Nissinen A, Vartiainen E. *The North Karelia Project. 20 Year results and experiences.* Helsinki: National Public Health Institute, 1995.

13 Taylor CB, Fortmann SP, Flora J, Kayman *et al.* Effect of long term community health education on body mass index: the Stanford Five City Project. *Am J Epidemiol* 1991:**134**;235–49.

14 Jeffery RW, Gray CW, French SA, Hellerstedt WL *et al.* Evaluation of weight reduction in a community intervention for cardiovascular disease risk: changes in body mass index in the Minnesota Heart Health Program. *Int J Obes Relat Metab Disord* 1995:**19**:30–35.

15 Food Standards Agency. *The balance of good health.* London: FSA, 2003.

16 NHS Centre for Reviews and Dissemination. *The prevention and treatment of childhood obesity.* Effective Healthcare Bulletins, vol 7, no 6. York: CRD, 2002.

17 Department for Education and Employment. *National Healthy School Standard: Guidance.* London: DfEE, 1999.

18 Department of Health. *Improvement, expansion and reform: priorities and planning framework 2003-06.* London: DH, 2002.

19 Maryon Davis A, Giles A, Rona R. *Tackling obesity: a toolbox for local partnership action.* London: Faculty of Public Health Medicine, 2000.

20 Baric L. The settings approach – implications for policy and strategy. *J Inst Health Educ* 1993:**31**(1):13–24.

21 Health Development Agency. *The management of obesity and overweight: an analysis of reviews of diet, physical activity and behavioural approaches.* London: HDA, 2003.

22 Hennrikus DJ, Jeffery RW. Worksite intervention for weight control: a review of the literature. *Am J Health Promot* 1996:**10**:471–98.

23 Shephard RJ. Worksite fitness and exercise programs: a review of methodology and health impact. *Am J Health Promot* 1996:**10**:436–52.

24 Harvey EL, Glenny A-M, Kirk SFL, Summerbell CD. Improving health professionals' management and the organisation of care for overweight and obese people (Cochrane Review). In: *The Cochrane Library*, Issue 2. Oxford: Update Software, 2001.

5 Health professionals: tackling overweight and obesity in the clinical setting

5.1   Proper nutritional care is fundamental to good clinical practice, as highlighted in a previous report of the Royal College of Physicians (RCP).[1] The RCP has also emphasised the importance of physical activity in preventing and controlling obesity.[2,3] There is a need for health professionals to develop and implement local nutritional care practice, policies, standards and audits based on national guidelines. This is important both for the promotion of healthy eating and an active lifestyle to prevent overweight and obesity in the public at large, and for the treatment of patients with overweight and obesity.

5.2   The main clinical setting for such educational and therapeutic strategies is usually primary care, but many of those at risk, or already overweight or obese, may be referred to secondary care. If the recommendations of this report are to be effectively implemented right across the health sectors, there is a need to engage all health professionals, irrespective of their discipline.

Setting standards

5.3   There should be increased emphasis on setting standards by which to judge the performance of local plans to tackle obesity. The medical royal colleges and other health professional organisations have a responsibility here. Examples of such standards are set out in the RCP publication, *Nutrition and patients – a doctor's responsibility*.[1] Standards for the management of overweight and obesity should be developed within a framework of clinical governance (see Box 5.1).

Training

5.4   The dramatic increase in the prevalence of overweight and obesity has not been matched by an increase in the amount of education and training provided for health professionals. Indeed, despite increasing pressure over the

---

Box 5.1 Nutritional clinical governance: recommendations to NHS trusts and primary care organisations/strategic health authorities.[1]

For the trust:

▶ The important role of nutritional care in the delivery of the NHS Plan and national service frameworks (eg CHD, older people's health and diabetes) should be recognised.

▶ For nutrition to have the status it deserves within trusts, the board should nominate a member as 'nutrition champion' and state its commitment to including nutritional care within the overall clinical governance framework.

▶ Each trust should establish a multiprofessional nutritional advisory group (or equivalent) with sufficient powers to oversee, coordinate and integrate agreed nutritional policies and practices into everyday patient care.

▶ Everyone – from kitchen staff to consultants – should have a clear understanding of roles and responsibilities in the provision of food, feeding and nutritional care.

▶ Nutritional care should be included in the trust's strategy and structure for clinical governance and audit.

▶ The trust should provide sufficient resources for proper clinical governance of nutritional care.

▶ The trust should be able to respond positively to sound cases made by clinical teams for service changes arising from a clinical governance approach.

▶ Patient advocacy and liaison services should be fully engaged in the above arrangements.

For primary care organisations and strategic health authorities/boards:

▶ Clinical governance of nutritional care should be incorporated into service level agreements (or equivalent) with trusts and primary care practices.

▶ Standards should include an appropriate level of dietetic support for primary care, particularly with regard to undernutrition, diabetes, obesity, and hyperlipidaemia.

▶ Nutritional care must comprise a key element of the performance assessment of trusts and primary care, and be conducted in sufficient depth and detail to learn useful practical lessons.

▶ Health authorities/boards have a role in sharing good practice with regard to nutritional care.

---

past decade to expand the nutrition and physical activity elements in the core training of doctors, nurses, pharmacists and allied health professionals, these subjects remain poorly addressed. Comprehensive training in the promotion of healthy eating, an active lifestyle and behaviour change should be provided at every level.

5.5   Too often health professionals ignore the obvious signs or symptoms of a nutritional disorder in patients and, if they are overweight, simply instruct them to go on a diet. It is therefore not surprising that interventions are only used after medical complications have become apparent. This oversight reflects a poor understanding of nutritional issues and a lack of knowledge and skills about their management. There is limited information provided in both undergraduate and postgraduate training programmes and scant coverage in specialist medical training. The medical profession's lack of appreciation of the medical consequences of obesity is reflected in the absence of specialist units in most regional hospitals and a reluctance to consider medication or surgery for patients most at risk. Since clinical teachers have had little or no training in clinical nutrition, they tend not to teach it.

> **Box 5.2 Recommendations for training at undergraduate, postgraduate and post-registration level.**
>
> *Undergraduate or pre-registration training*
> ▸ Every opportunity should be taken to introduce nutritional concepts into undergraduate training.
> ▸ Nutrition is a key component of health and illness and should be recognised as such by students.
> ▸ Students should be engaged with the science and application of nutrition because good nutritional principles should be followed by themselves.
> ▸ Students need to understand the multiple health benefits of physical activity.
>
> *Postgraduate or advanced training and continuing professional development*
> ▸ Health professionals should be motivated to regard the nutrition/exercise balance ('energy in' and 'energy out') as important in the prevention and management of disease and the promotion of good health.
> ▸ Regular multi-professional teaching sessions on obesity, nutrition and physical activity should be included as part of training programmes – this should include guidance on nutritional assessment (including body fat), the nutritional and exercise requirements in health and disease, and an appreciation of poor nutrition and a lack of exercise as determinants of risk.
> ▸ The prevention and management of overweight and obesity may be divided within a modular training programme to enable health professionals to gain knowledge and skills in a stepwise manner.
> ▸ Health professionals should be trained to facilitate behaviour change in their patients while remaining sensitive to the complex social and emotional issues surrounding obesity.

5.6   The implementation of education and training will necessarily involve universities, training colleges for professions allied to medicine, nursing and medical schools, postgraduate medical institutions, the National Health Service University (NHSU) and the medical royal colleges.

5.7   Research has highlighted the limited confidence of nurses and dietetics staff in assisting patients with their attempts to lose weight. Family doctors often fail to recognise obesity as a serious medical condition and commonly recommend weight management only when an accompanying comorbidity is evident. Research also suggests a very negative approach to the obese, with many health professionals believing its management to be frustrating, time-consuming and pointless.[1]

5.8   Health professionals should better understand the causes and consequences of increasing body fatness and appreciate the importance of prevention and intervention where the condition is established. They should also be able to recognise a familial tendency to overweight and obesity and bear the family history in mind when managing the individual patient. Importantly, management must be sensitive to the feelings of those with the condition and demonstrate appropriate attitudes towards them.

References

1   Royal College of Physicians. *Nutrition and patients – a doctor's responsibility*. Report of a working party. London: RCP, 2002.
2   Royal College of Physicians. *Medical aspects of exercise*. London: RCP, 1991.
3   Royal College of Physicians. *Physical activity for patients: an exercise prescription*. London: RCP, 2001.